New Pharmacological and Epidemiological Data in Analgesics Research

Edited by
K. Brune

1990

Springer Basel AG

Editor's Address:
Prof. Dr. K. Brune
Institut für Pharmakologie und Toxikologie der Universität Erlangen-Nürnberg
Universitätsstraße 22
D–8520 Erlangen, FRG

Copy-Editing by Dr. J.C.F. Habicht, D–6915 Dossenheim, FRG

ISBN 978-3-7643-2452-0   ISBN 978-3-0348-6387-2 (eBook)
DOI 10.1007/978-3-0348-6387-2
Deutsche Bibliothek Cataloging-in-Publication Data

New pharmacological and epidemiological data in analgesics research / ed. by K. Brune. –
Basel ; Boston ; Berlin : Birkhäuser, 1990

NE: Brune, Kay [Hrsg.]

Contents

Preface

More than 100 years ago, in 1884, the first fully synthetic drug, phenazone, was discovered and introduced into therapy. It proved to possess both antipyretic and analgesic properties. To date, phenazone and many of its derivatives continue to be used extensively to relieve pain, fever and discomfort. This group of drugs, however, was not readily accepted in anglo-saxon countries because early estimates indicated a relatively high risk of agranulocytosis. Moreover, the early discovery and extensive use of these compounds prohibited both an exact definition of their mode of action and the realization of double-blind controlled studies proving the compounds' analgesic effects according to modern standards. Both aspects led to a certain degree of dissatisfaction with the use of pyrazole drugs which was accompanied by public criticism and, in some parts of the world, restrictions on the use of the most popular and efficacious compound in this group, dipyrone.

Over the past ten years, however, impressive data on the safety of dipyrone, its performance in different experimental pain systems and new hints as to its mode of action have been carefully gathered by a small number of research groups. Their results are noteworthy in two respects. Firstly, the data from M. Levy and his colleagues have proved that dipyrone is not an absolutely safe drug. Its safety, however, is comparable to that of the best of the non-opioid analgesics currently available. Secondly, the studies by H.O. Handwerker, G. Kobal and R.F. Schmidt, initiated several years ago by myself, have demonstrated that dipyrone (metamizol) is a highly efficient analgesic without the pronounced anti-inflammatory effects typically observed with the aspirin-like compounds. Moreover, it has become clear that dipyrone exerts at least part of its analgesic action in the spinal cord, without the involvement of either aminergic or opioid receptors. Most of these results are compiled in this book.

In the light of this recent research, dipyrone presents itself as an interesting compound with a distinct mode of action which differs from that of the opioids and that of the aspirin-like drugs. In addition, it is devoid of the gastrointestinal toxicity of aspirin and ibuprofen as well as the addictiveness of the opiates and opioids. In other words, dipyrone is a compound which possesses many of the characteristics of the "ideal" pain-relieving agent which most laboratories involved in the development of new analgesics are still seeking to develop.

Prof. Dr. med. K. Brune
Erlangen, 1 January, 1990

New aspects of the mode of action of dipyrone

X. He, V. Neugebauer, H.-G. Schaible and R.F. Schmidt
Physiologisches Institut der Universität Würzburg
Röntgenring 9
D–8700 Würzburg, F.R.G.

The pyrazolone derivative, dipyrone (metamizol), is extensively employed in the treatment of acute and chronic pain and of inflammatory processes. The drug is a potent analgesic agent with some antipyretic, anti-inflammatory and spasmolytic properties. It is often classified as peripherally acting since it is rapidly metabolized into 4-methylaminoantipyrine and 4-aminoantipyrine which have both been shown to have a potency to inhibit prostaglandin synthesis similar to that of acetylsalicylic acid (ASA). However, this matter has never been fully clarified, and there are some indications in the literature that metamizol also has a central site of action [1][2].

In regard to the peripheral site of action, it is difficult to understand why there is such a wide discrepancy between the very strong analgesic action of dipyrone on the one hand and its rather weak anti-inflammatory action on the other. Two hypotheses have mainly been advanced to explain this discrepancy. 1) A differential influence of the various peripherally acting analgesic drugs on cyclo-oxygenase, depending on the type of tissue from which the cyclo-oxygenase is being released; it is presumed that the analgesic acids inhibit prostaglandin synthesis mainly in the periphery and particularly in inflamed tissue, whereas the non-acidic compounds inhibit mainly in the central nervous system. 2) It has been postulated that dipyrone has a central site of action in the periaquaeductal grey (PAG) by activating descending inhibitory pathways at this site [3][4].

To elucidate the action of metamizol further and to detect, in particular, any differential action of metamizol on the one hand and antiphlogistic algesics like aspirin (ASA) and indomethacin on the other, we investigated the effect of these drugs in our model of acute experimental arthritis in the knee-joint of the cat. In a first series of experiments we tested the influence of dipyrone on the discharge behaviour of fine afferent nerve fibres innervating an acutely inflamed joint. Preceeding experiments under these conditions in our laboratory had already shown that acetylsalicylic acid and indomethacin had a significant effect on the resting activity and on the movement-evoked activity of fine myelinated group III (Aδ) and unmyelinated group IV C afferent units [5]. Similarly, under the same circumstances, opiates have been shown to exert inhibitory effects on spontaneous discharges in small-diameter afferents from inflamed knee-joints in the cat [6]. In a second series of experiments the spinal inhibitory action of dipyrone was tested. These recordings were made from ascending tract cells in the spinal cords of anaesthetized spinalized cats after acute arthritis was induced in the knee-joint [7][8].

Remarks on methods

All experiments were performed with adult cats anaesthetized initially by intramuscular injection of 15 mg/kg ketamine hydrochloride followed by i.v. injection of 60 mg/kg α-chloralose. Additional doses of chloralose (10–20 mg/kg i.v.) were given as required to maintain a deep level of anaesthesia. All animals were immobilized with pancuronium bromide (Pancuronium, Organon) 0.6 mg/h i.v. and artificially ventilated. Blood pressure, end-expiratory CO_2 and body temperature were monitored and kept at physiological levels.

The techniques used in the peripheral experiments, i.e. the dissection of the right leg, the setting-up of the animal on the mounting table and the performance of passive limb movements, have previously been described in detail [9][10][11].

For the spinal experiments the lower thoracic and lumbosacral spinal cord was exposed by laminectomy from T12 to L7. The cord was transected in the lower thoracic region after injection of approx. 0.1 ml of procaine hydrochloride (10 mg/ml) at the level of interruption to prevent mechanical activation of axons in the long spinal tracts. The spinal roots and denticulate ligaments at T13 to L1 were cut so that the spinal cord could be mounted on a pair of platinum stimulating electrodes. The dorsal funiculi were interrupted by crushing them with forceps just caudal to the stimulating electrodes to prevent orthodromic activation of tract cells by volleys descending in axons of the dorsal columns. The spinal cord was covered with warm mineral oil in a pool bounded by skin flaps. Recordings were made from ascending tract cells using carbon filament microelectodes. Unitary activity was displayed on an oscilloscope. At the same time, the action potentials were fed into a window discriminator, and standard pulses triggered by them were used by a digital computer to generate single pass peristimulus time histograms. The action potentials and the pulses were also stored on magnetic tape for further off-line analysis.

In both series of experiments an acute inflammation of the knee-joint was induced early in the experiments. This was accomplished by injecting first kaolin (4%, 0.3–0.5 ml) and then, 15 min. later, carrageenan (2% 0.3 ml) into the knee-joint cavity. Either of these substances induces acute inflammation, but their combined use appears to cause a greater degree of inflammation with a more consistent time course than does the individual agent. Flexion and extension movements were repeated for a period of 5 min. following the kaolin and the carrageenan injection in this series of experiments.

Effect of experimental arthritis on the discharge characteristics of primary afferents and spinal neurons

The major effects of the experimental arthritis on the discharge behaviour of primary afferents and of spinal cord neurons can be summarized as follows [7][8][11][12].

The arthritis increased mechanosensitivity in the majority of low-threshold units, i.e. in units that even in the normal joint responded to movements in the working range. The augmentation of reactions in most cases developed within the first hour after the injection of the inflammatory compounds, sometimes starting immediately after the injection. A further rise in the mechanosensitivity was observed within the following 2–4 h. In most group III units enhanced responses to movements were accompanied by an induction of or increase in spontaneous discharges.

More importantly, the inflammation led to enhanced mechanosensitivity in high-threshold afferents, i.e., in units that in the normal joint responded only to noxious movements exeeding the working range of the knee. In most units these changes occurred within the second to third hour after the induction of inflammation, with a further increase occuring later on. In a high proportion of these units resting activity was also induced. The experimental arthritis also induced afferent activity in fine afferents that in the normal joint were unresponsive to local mechanical stimulation and to movement («waking up» of «sleeping» nociceptors). The time course of these changes was similar to that in high-threshold fibres. In summary, these results show that acute experimental arthritis leads to enhanced mechanosensitivity in various types of articular afferents including non-nociceptive as well as nociceptive and initially unresponsive ones.

In the spinal experiments the neurons were found in segments L4–L7 in spinal cord and in various laminae. All of the units had a convergent input from the knee-joint and from other tissue, such as skin or muscle. Responses to flexion of the knee, an innocuous stimulus, were recorded before and several hours after the injection of kaolin and carrageenan. The results were as follows. Nociceptive-specific neurons without responses to innocuous movement in the normal joint started to respond to such movements when the joint was becoming inflamed. Significant reactions commenced within the second or third hour after induction of inflammation and the size of the responses increased progressively. Wide-dynamic-range neurons with responses to innocuous movements of the knee even prior to inflammation showed enhanced reactions in the course of the arthritis. Thus, arthritis significantly modifies the discharges of different types of spinal neurons with joint input. As the neurons under study had ascending axons and the time course of the changes in responsiveness matched the behavioural changes in conscious, freely moving cats, such neurons may contribute to the central mechanisms which during acute arthritis lead to the sensation of pain and/or the corresponding «pain reactions» (pseudaffective responses).

Effect of dipyrone on the resting activity of fine afferents from inflamed joints

Effect on group III afferents. The action of dipyrone (metamizol) on a group III unit (conduction velocity 8.0 m/s) from an inflamed joint is shown in Fig.1. In a control period of 40 min. the resting activity was rather stable around 71.9 ± 15.6 imp/min. (Fig. 1A and first histogram in B). Thereafter, dipyrone (25mg/kg body weight) was given intravenously. As shown in diagram A in Fig. 1, it takes approx. 20 min. before any tendency towards a decrease in resting activity can be seen. 60–68 min. after the injection (Fig. 1B, second histogram from above) the resting activity was reduced to 51.9 ± 5.3 imp/s. 110–118 min. after the injection (Fig. 1B, third histogram from above) the resting activity was only 32.4 ± 6.9 imp/min. At this time the resting activity reached its lowest level, and, as compared to the control activity, it was also much more regular. No recovery from this effect of metamizol could be observed for up to 260 min. after the administration of dipyrone.

Altogether, 10 group III fibres were investigated in this way, all of them showing a similar decrease in their spontaneous activity. The average resting activity of these 10 fibres during the control period was 103.3 ± 80.3 imp/min. After metamizol the impulse fequency was reduced to 75.4 ± 61.2 imp/min. Using the t-test it was shown that in 7 of the 10 fibres there was a high significance $p<1\%$, in one fibre the significance was $(5\%>p>1\%)$, and in the two other fibres the difference in activity before and after the administration of dipyrone was not significant.

From these results it is concluded that dipyrone has a definite inhibitory action on the spontaneous activity of group III afferent units from inflamed joints. In most cases the decrease in resting discharge became significant 21–30 min. after the administration of dipyrone. In the following 1–4 h after administration no recovery from this depression could be observed.

Action of dipyrone on the resting activity of group IV afferent units. In contrast to the results with group III fibres those with group IV units were not unequivocal. Five of the 10 group IV units (conduction velocities <2.5 m/s) even showed a certain rise in frequency under dipyrone. In the other fibres the averages of spontaneous activity fell below the control level. However, in three of the fibres, this decrease did not reach a level of significance. These results show that

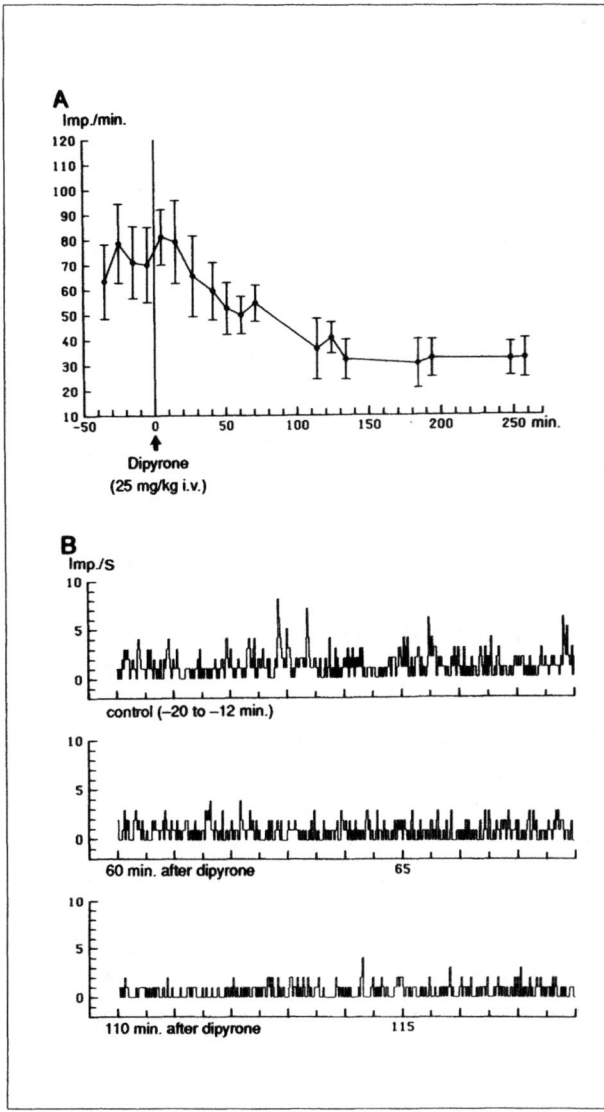

Fig. 1.
Resting activity of a group III unit (conduction velocity 8.0 m/s) before and after i.v. administration of 25 mg/kg body weight dipyrone.
A. Means and standard deviations of the number of impulses/min. in 10-min. periods. B. Three sections of the continuous registration of the peristimulus time histogram. The address advance time was 1 s. From [13].

metamizol does not reduce the discharge rates of inflamed group IV articular afferent units from the knee-joint of the cat. In other words, the results indicate that dipyrone exerts peripheral analgesic action which is exclusively or mainly restricted to the fine myelinated units.

Spinal antinociceptive effect of dipyrone

The rather restricted effect dipyrone has on the discharges of primary afferent units from inflamed joints indicates that the strong analgesic action this drug exhibits in pain patients most probably is not exclusively due to its peripheral action. On the contrary, it appears most likely that additional central sites of action are responsible for the drug's powerful analgesic effects. To elucidate this central mechanism further, the experiments described below were performed in spinal cats.

As briefly outlined above and published in detail elsewhere [8], both noci-ceptive-specific and wide-dynamic-range neurons with ascending axons and input from the knee-joint display considerable modifications of their spontaneous and evoked discharge behaviour in the course of experimental arthritis. The large amplification of their spontaneous and evoked responses under such conditions is a direct consequence of the considerable amplification of the primary afferent input induced by the experimental arthritis. In addition, we have also observed that local interneurons as well as motoneurons show a similar increase in their discharges [14]. These effects of inflammation on the responses of spinal neurons appear to serve as a useful neural model of the events responsible for the development of arthritic pain.

The effects of dipyrone on the discharges of spinal neurons are ex-emplified in Fig. 2. This neuron had its localization in lamina VIII and an axon projecting up the spinal cord. Under control conditions it displayed some resting activity (left-hand side in Fig. 2). After articular inflammation the resting activity increased to several times the control level. As shown in the figure, the intravenous injection of dipyrone 50 mg/kg reduced this spon-taneous activity by more than 50% of the preinjection value within the first 10 min. after injection, and there was some further decline in the subsequent hour. Actually, within 1 h the resting activity returned to the control values (right-hand side in Fig. 2).

Similar results were obtained in practically all other units tested in this way. In additon, the unit shown in Fig. 2, and many others, also showed considerable decrease in the discharges evoked by flexion and/or extension of the joint, and by stimulation of the receptive fields in the skin and muscle outside the articular tissue.

A summary of the results from 11 neurons tested consecutively in this way is shown in Fig. 3. As seen in A, most units showed a decrease in their resting activity (RA) as well as their evoked activity (EA). In some units the depressant effect was restricted either to the evoked or the resting activity, and in a further two units no effect of dipyrone could be observed.

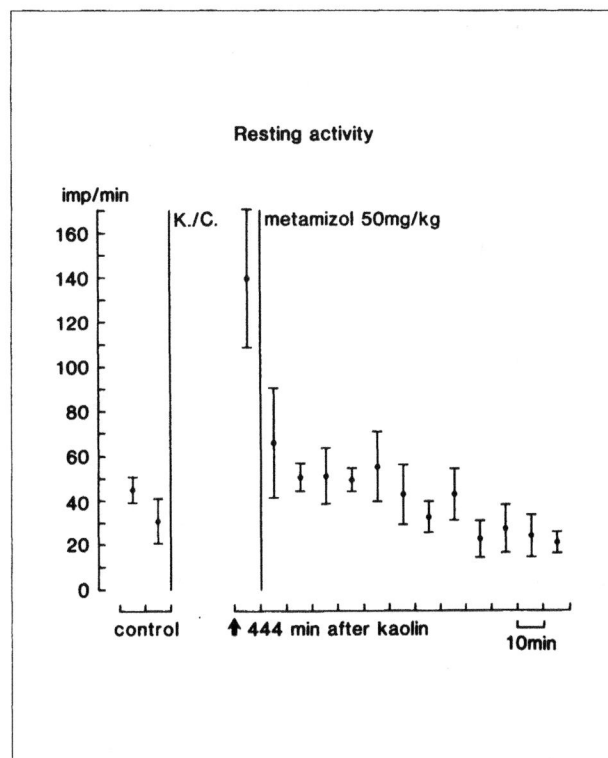

Fig. 2.
Effects of dipyrone (metamizol) 50 mg/kg (i.v.) on the resting activity of a spinal laminae VIII neuron with an axon projecting to supraspinal areas. The unit was of the wide-dynamic-range type having receptive fields in the skin, deep tissue and knee-joint. The drug was injected 444 min. after induction of inflammation by kaolin followed by carrageenan (see «Remarks on methods»). The graph shows means and standard deviations of consecutive 10-min. periods. Note the rapid decline in impulse frequency following dipyrone injection. There was a slower decline to the control level in the following 60 min.

It is interesting to note that the onset of the effect of dipyrone on the resting discharges was always within less than 10 min. after injection (Fig. 1B). This time course is considerably faster than that observed for the reduction of the afferent discharges of group III units (Fig. 1). Therefore, it is extremely unlikely that the spinal effects of the drug are a consequence of a change in primary afferent input.

The onset of the changes in evoked activity was somewhat slower than in the case of the resting activity (Fig. 3C). Again, in two units the effects were clearly visible within the first 10 min. after injection, but for the other units the effects could only be seen within 15–25 min. after injecting dipyrone. The extent of the changes in the evoked responses is not illustrated here, but it may be said that it is even more impressive in many cases than that occurring with the spontaneous discharges.

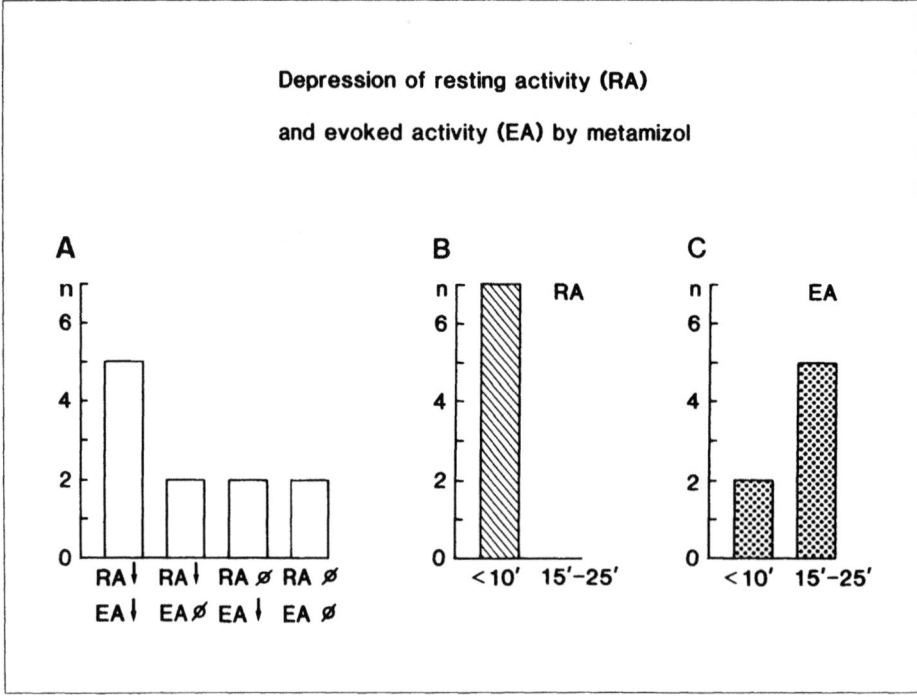

Fig. 3.
The effect of dipyrone (metamizol) on the resting activity (RA) and evoked activity (EA) of
11 spinal neurons recorded consecutively. A. A depressant effect of the drug was observed
in 9 of the 11 neurons. In 5 cells both the evoked activity and the resting activity were
depressed. In two cells only the resting activity and in two other cells only the evoked activity
showed reduction. B. The reduction in resting activity always began within the first 10 min.
after drug administration. C. Time of onset of the effect on evoked activity.

Concluding remarks

In the present experiments both the peripheral and the spinal effects of dipyrone
on the resting and evoked discharges of primary afferent units and of ascending
neurons and spinal interneurons were investigated under the conditions of acute
experimental arthritis in the knee-joint of the cat. The results presented indicate
that dipyrone causes antinociceptive effects and analgesia not only by peripheral
action on low- and high-threshold fine myelinated afferents but also by a central
effect which must clearly be directed at the spinal cord, because the experiments
were conducted in acutely spinalized cats. No effect was seen on the discharge
behaviour of unmyelinated group IV units (C fibres), and the effects on the group

III units (Aδ delta units) were small. It is, therefore, postulated that the analgesic action of dipyrone is mainly due to its central effects. As outlined in the introduction, these central sites of action may not only include the spinal cord but also extend to other central sites such as the periaquaeductal grey (PAG). These differential effects of dipyrone could easily explain the otherwise puzzling finding that the drug's strong analgesic action is not matched by an equally potent anti-inflammatory effect.

References

1. Driesen, W., Hahn, F., Rummel, W. (1950): Über den Einfluss von Cardiazol, Coramin und Pyramidon auf das Elektroencephalogramm (E.E.G.) und das Myeologramm von Katzen und Kaninchen, Dtsch. Z. Nervenheilk. *164*, 395–406.

2. Starkenstein, E., Hendrych, F. und Escobar-Bordoy, J. (1934): Zur experimentellen Analyse der Pyramidonwirkung. Naunyn-Schmiedebergs Arch. exp. Path. Pharmak. *176*, 486–493.

3. Carlsson, K.-H., Helmreich, J., Jurna, I. (1986): Activation of inhibition from the periaqueductal grey matter mediates central analgesic effects of metamizol (dipyrone) Pain *27*, 373–390.

4. Carlsson, K.-H., Jurna, I. (1987): The role of descending inhibition in the antinociceptive effects of the pyrazolone derivates, metamizol (dipyrone) and aminophenazone («Pyramidon»). Naunyn-Schmiedeberg's Archives of Pharmacology *335*, 154–159.

5. Heppelmann, B., Pfeffer, A., Schaible, H.-G., Schmidt, R.F. (1986): Effects of acetylsalicylic acid and indomethacin on single groups III and IV sensory units from acutely inflamed joints. Pain *26*, 337–351.

6. Russell, N.J.W., Schaible, H.-G., Schmidt, R.F. (1987): Opiates inhibit the discharges of fine afferent units from inflamed knee-joint of the cat. Neurosc. Letters *76*, 107–112.

7. Schaible, H.-G., Schmidt, R.F., Willis, W.D. (1987a): Convergent inputs from articular, cutaneous and muscle receptors onto ascending tract cells in the cat spinal cord. Exp. Brain Research *66*, 479–488.

8. Schaible, H.-G., Schmidt, R.F., Willis, W.D. (1987b): Enhancement of the response of ascending tract cells in the cat spinal cord by acute inflammation of the knee-joint. Exp. Brain Research *66*, 489–499.

9.. Schaible, H.-G., Schmidt, R.F. (1983a): Activation of groups III and IV sensory units in medial articular nerve by mechanical stimulation of knee-joint. J. Neurophysiol. *49*, 35–44.

10. Schaible, H.-G., Schmidt, R.F. (1983b): Responses of fine medial articular nerve afferents to passive movements of knee-joint. J. Neurophysiol. *49*, 1118–1126.

11. Schaible, H.-G., Schmidt, R.F. (1985): Effects of an experimental arthritis on the sensory properties of fine articular afferent units. J. Neurophysiol. *54*, 1109–1122.

12. Schaible, H.-G., Schmidt, R.F. (1988): Time course of mechanosensitivity changes in articular afferents during a developing experimental arthritis. J. Neurophysiol. *60*, 2180–2195.
     Schaible, H.-G., Schmidt, R.F., Willis, W.D. (1986): Responses of spinal cord neurones to stimulation of articular afferent fibres in the cat. J. Physiol. (Lond) *372*, 575–593.

13. He, X. (1987): Wirkung von Metamizol auf die Ruheaktivität der Gruppe III und Gruppe IV Fasern des N. Articularis Medialis im akut experimentell enzündeten Kniegelenk der Katze.

Promotionsschrift, Medizinische Fakultät der Bayerischen Julius-Maximilians-Universität, Würzburg.

14. He, X., Proske, U., Schaible, H.-G., Schmidt, R.F. (1988): Acute inflammation of the knee-joint in the cat alters responses of flexor motoneurons to leg movements. J. Neurophysiol. *59*, 326–340.

Analgesic effects of dipyrone as compared to placebo

H.O. Handwerker, A. Beck, C. Forster, Th. Gall and W. Magerl
Institut für Physiologie und Biokybernetik
der Universität Erlangen
Universitätsstraße 17
D–8520 Erlangen, F.R.G.

Introduction

In theory, experimental algesimetry models seem to offer advantages for measuring the potency of analgesic drugs over clinical observations, where the assessment of analgesia is often influenced by illness-related variables. In particular, it should be easier to relate the time course of the analgesic effect to the kinetics of the drugs, since stimuli can be applied in a planned manner. However, in spite of their theoretical superiority, the usefullness of experimental studies on healthy subjects for measuring drug effects is still controversial. The assessment of the effects of non-opioid analgesics with those methods provides exceptional difficulties, probably due to their minor psychotropic effects.

According to Beecher's classic studies [1][2] these problems are mainly due to the fact that experimental pain stimuli are often unrealistic models of clinical pain. Indeed, an experimental study on volunteers always has to avoid significant injury. Hence, of the three major dimensions of pain [3] the sensory dimension is prominent in experimental situations, compared with the affective and evaluative dimensions. This classical critique of experimental algesimetry may still apply to its use for the study of narcotic analgesics. The problems encountered with non-narcotic drugs may have additional reasons which only recently became comprehensible with the progress of basic research on pain mechanisms.

Nowadays it has been established that the nociceptors undergo sensitization processes in the course of inflammation that induces spontaneous discharges and changes their responsiveness to chemical and physical stimuli. In turn the increased nociceptor input to the central nervous system seems to induce plasticity changes in ascending pathways [4]. Non-narcotic analgesic drugs apparently diminish or prevent sensitization at peripheral and/or central sites. The time-honoured distinction between «centrally» and «peripherally» acting analgesics has to be re-evaluated in the light of newer insights into the plasticity of the nociceptive system.

For that reason we have attempted to develop an algesimetric technique which meets two demands: (a) the stimuli have to sensitize nociceptors, and (b) the method has to allow the assessment of several parameters of the drug action which represent the activity of the nociceptor system at different levels of integration.

This technique has been employed in a placebo-controlled double-blind study on the effects of dipyrone, ibuprofen and paracetamol. The complete study will be published elsewhere, but some of the findings on dipyrone are reported in this paper.

Methods

Design of the stimulus

The experimental design was modified from that used successfully by our group to demonstrate the analgesic effect of acetylsalicylic acid [5][6].

Pain was induced by alternatingly pinching two interdigital webs of the left hand with a feedback-controlled stimulator. Each stimulus lasted 2 min. Stimuli were applied at 10-min. intervals; i.e. each of the two stimulated skin areas were pinched at intervals of 20 min. To induce two levels of pain we pinched the web between the 2nd and 3rd finger with 10 N and the web between 3rd and 4th finger with 8 N (at 28 mm^2). With these stimuli, pain described as aching and throbbing was induced; it increased slowly during each stimulus (see Fig. 1) and in the course of the experiment (see Fig. 2). The increased painfulness may indicate nociceptor sensitization.

Assessment of pain-related parameters

As in the previous studies [5][6] the subjects rated their current pain level at 10-s intervals throughout each stimulus, following acoustic signals. Ratings were performed by moving a lever which controlled the display of a visual analogue scale (VAS) on a computer screen. The end points of the VAS were defined as «no pain» and «tolerance limit».

Previously we have found that our pain stimuli induced a reflex vasoconstriction in the skin of the stimulated hand outlasting each stimulus for 1 min. or more [7]. This nocifensive reflex is mediated by sympathetic vasoconstrictor efferents and may provide a parameter of the processing of the nociceptive input at the spinal and brainstem level. In this study we have assessed the vasoconstriction with finger-photoplethysmography (FPP) and with computer-supported infrared thermography.

FPP from the thumb reflected quick changes in skin blood flow readily. The output of this device consists of electrical conduction changes in a photo-resistor induced by backscattered light [8]. Unfortunately it cannot be calibrated in terms of absolute blood flow. We maintained comparability between sessions by keeping the impedance bridge calibrated. The technique will be described in detail elsewhere (Geldner, Magerl, Handwerker, in prep.). Thermography provides absolute measures of the skin surface temperature. For the purpose of this study thermographic images of the hand were obtained at 30-s intervals. The mean temperature of the 2nd finger was computed for assessing the reflex magnitude. Comparison of FPP- and thermography-derived parameters improves the interpretation of skin blood flow changes assessed with both devices.

After the first stimuli a flare appeared around the stimulated site which became visible in thermography as an area which was warmer than the rest of the hand. This vasodilation developed more slowly than the reflex vasoconstriction and was assessed by subtracting the mean temperature in the erythematous area from that in a reference area at the hypothenar [7]. Since no such flare was observed after a chronic nerve lesion (Magerl, unpublished observations) we assume that this inflammatory reaction is at least partly mediated by the release of vasoactive substances, probably neuropeptides, from the stimulated nociceptors. In that case it represents a «neurogenic», nociceptor-mediated inflammatory reaction.

In summary, the impact of the analgesic drugs was assessed on three reaction levels: that of the local inflammatory response, that of the sympathetic reflex, and that of the conscious pain experience.

Experimental protocol

The experiment was designed as a double-blind cross-over study with 22 subjects (12 male and 10 female, age 24–33 years). Each subject participated in one practice and four medication sessions. The only purpose of the praxis session was to familiarize the subjects with the experimental procedure. Seven to ten days elapsed from session to session.

The experimental sessions started at 8.00 a.m. with a standardized breakfast. At 9.30 the subject swallowed two equal-looking capsules containing either placebo, 1000 mg dipyrone, 800 mg ibuprofen, or 1000 mg paracetamol, with 100 ml of water. The first 8-N stimulus was delivered 30 min. after drug intake, then 10-N and 8-N stimuli followed alternately. The last (12th) stimulus was applied after 140 min.

Ninty minutes after drug intake blood was taken by venous puncture. The plasma levels of the respective metabolites were assessed by HPLC in the

Department of Pharmacology, Erlangen (Prof. Brune). In the case of dipyrone all subjects had plasma levels of the four most important metabolites (4-aminoantipy-rine, 4-methylaminoantipyrine, 4-formylaminoantipyrine and 4-acetylaminoan-tipyrine) which were sufficient to preclude inadequate absorption.

The subjects were informed about the purpose of the study and the nature of the drugs. They were not explicitly informed, however, that a placebo was included.

The study was approved by the Ethics Committee of the Medical Faculty of the University of Erlangen. The subjects were told that they were free to withdraw from the experiment at any time.

Results

Pain ratings

The main focus of the study was on the impact of dipyrone (and other non-opioid analgesics) on the hyperalgesia and other signs of nociceptor sensitization induced (a) by the long duration of the individual stimuli and (b) by the stimulus repetition.

(a) We have previously shown that noxious mechanical stimuli become more and more painful over two minutes. This increasing painfulness is not due to increasing nociceptor discharges, and is hence probably a central phenomenon [9].

The average time course of the pain ratings in the placebo and dipyrone sessions is shown in Fig.1 for the six 10-N stimuli.

Higher pain ratings were obtained during stimuli applied later in the placebo sessions as compared to the responses obtained under dipyrone. However, there was obviously no faster increase of painfulness within a stimulus, but rather a parallel shift of the time courses. For the subsequent analyses we have therefore used the average rating of a subject in each trial as response parameter.

(b) The average pain responses to both 8-N and 10-N stimuli are shown in Fig. 2.

Apart from the two first 8-N and 10-N stimuli and the last (11th) 8-N stimulus the differences between placebo and dipyrone were always significant (paired t-test). It is obvious that stimulus repetition at the same site became increasingly painful under placebo, but not under dipyrone. It is also obvious that dipyrone did not affect the painfulness of stimuli delivered at the beginning of a session to previously untouched skin.

These results led us to conclude that two parameters derived from the pain ratings may best represent the hyperalgesia developing in a session and its prevention by dipyrone: the average responses during the later stimuli and the slope of the regression lines through the data sets shown in Fig. 2. Hence, for each

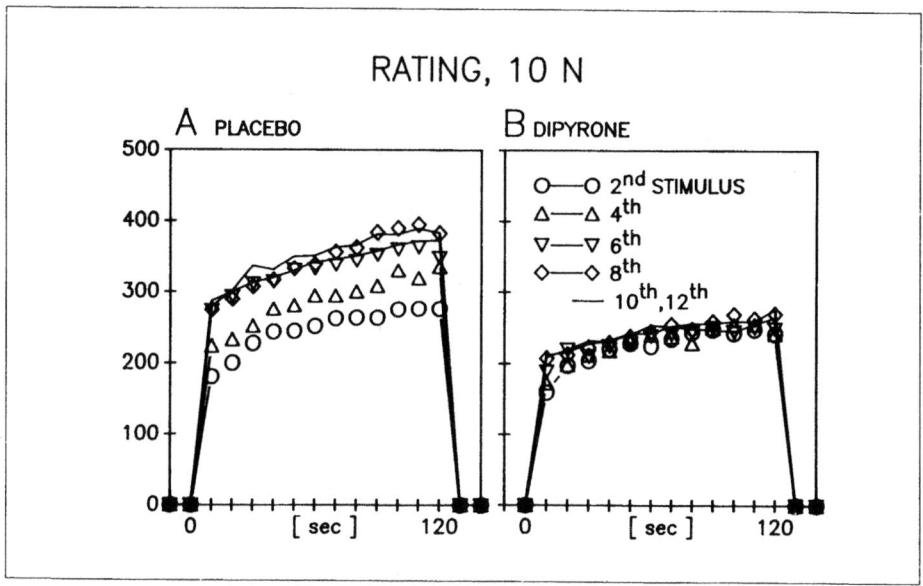

Fig. 1.
Mean pain ratings of 21 subjects during repeated 10-N stimulation in the placebo (A) and in the dipyrone (B) session. Ordinate: mean ratings in per mill of the visual analogue scale.

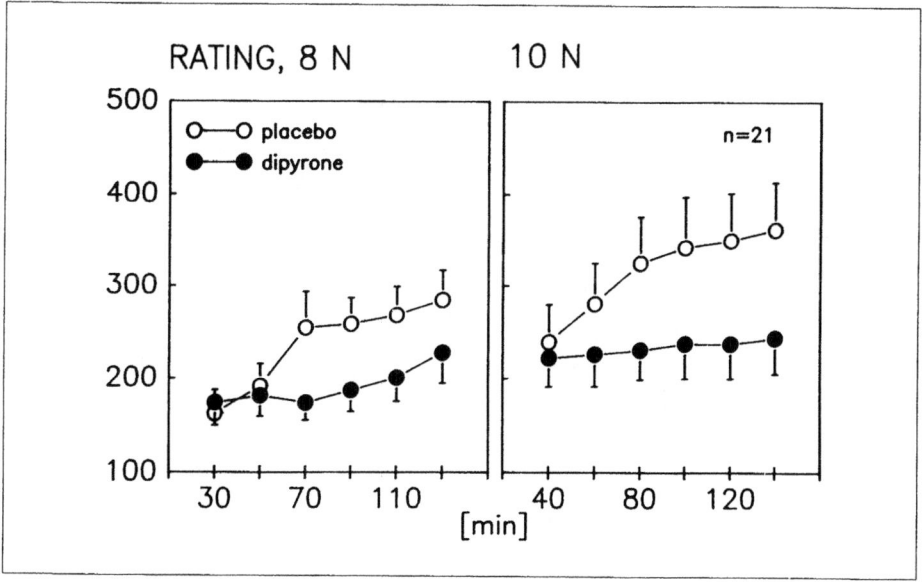

Fig. 2.
Time course of the average pain ratings during 8-N and 10-N stimuli under placebo and dipyrone. The symbols represent average responses obtained during individual stimuli of two minutes' duration. Error bars: SEM.

subject average ratings were computed for the 4-N, later 8-N, and 10-N stimuli (i.e. for the stimulus strength of 8-N the average ratings at the 5th, 7th, 9th and 11th stimulus, and for the stimulus strength of 10-N those of the 6th, 8th, 10th and 12th stimulus). The linear regression was computed for each subject from the whole data set which is also shown in Fig. 2.

The results of this data reduction are shown in Fig. 3.

The dipyrone effect is clearly reflected in both parameters. The slope of the regression line may be of particular interest, since it is not dependent on stimulus strength.

Sympathetic reflexes and local vasodilation

The FPP signal became progressively smaller throughout the experimental sessions under both placebo and dipyrone conditions. In parallel, the thermography revealed a slow drop in the skin temperature. This indicates vasoconstriction which is probably due to the long immobilization of the arm; this could not be avoided, even though the support for the hand was temperature-controlled. However, under placebo a significantly smaller FPP signal and a lower temperature were observed than in the dipyrone sessions, as well as in the control period of 30 s before each stimulus, at the peak of the reflex, and one minute after each stimulus (Fig. 4).

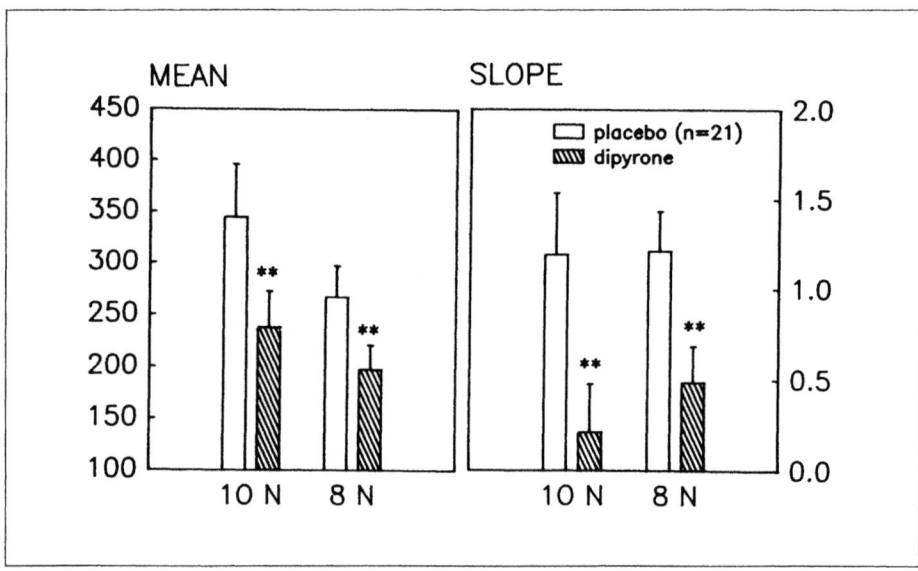

Fig. 3.
Comparison of the pain magnitude during the later stimuli in a session (mean) and of the increase in pain ratings throughout a session (slope) under placebo and dipyrone. Error bars: SEM. For further details see text.

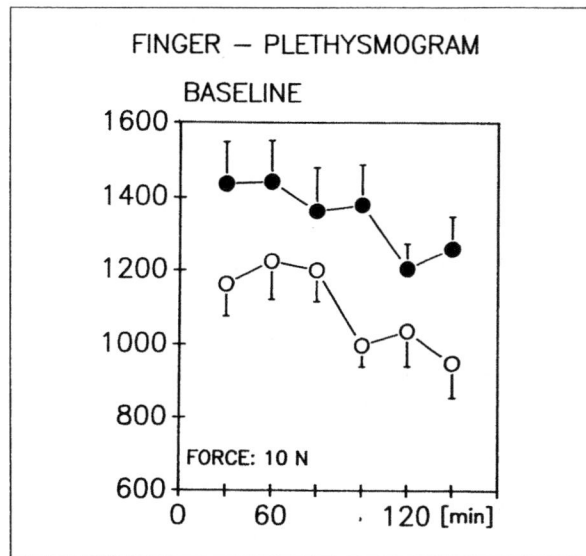

Fig. 4.
Baseline finger-photoplethys-mogram values measured im-mediately before 10-N stimuli under placebo (open circles) and dipyrone (closed dots). Error bars: SEM.

When the reflex measures were subtracted from the baseline, the differences between the two conditions were no longer significant. Hence, dipyrone not so much influences the amplitude of the reflex vasoconstriction, but rather induces tonic peripheral vasodilation. This interpretation fits with the well-known relaxant effects of dipyrone on smooth muscle cells.

Dipyrone did not significantly influence vasodilation in the skin surrounding the stimulated area. This parameter was, however, affected by ibuprofen.

Discussion

We report the analgesic effect of dipyrone on the pain responses of healthy subjects to pain induced by the pinching of a skin fold. The decrease in the pain ratings under dipyrone was highly significant. Moreover, dipyrone had the strongest analgesic effect of the three non-narcotic analgesic agents tested in this study.

However, a closer view reveals that the ratings in response to the first stimuli delivered in a session were not affected by dipyrone; only those to stimuli applied one hour or more after drug intake were. This was certainly not due to slow absorption of dipyrone, but rather reflected the fact that this drug mainly reduced the hyperalgesia induced by repeated stimulation of the same skin site. A similar result was obtained in a previous study on acetylsalicylic acid [6]. These findings demonstrate quite clearly that this group of agents acts predominantly by reducing the sensitized state of the nociceptive system.

Another aim of this study was to obtain information on the site of action of dipyrone by assessing several stimulus-induced reaction parameters that may represent different levels of integration in the nociceptive system.

Dipyrone had no impact on vasodilation in the skin surrounding the stimulus site. This negative finding seems to indicate that the drug did not exert any prominent anti-inflammatory action in our model, and this is in agreement with its weak anti-inflammatory actions in other models.

Nociceptive processing at the spinal/brainstem level was assessed by measuring the stimulus-induced reflex vasoconstriction in the stimulated hand. However, to our surprise dipyrone had a significant effect on the basal blood flow and hence the reflex amplitudes could not be properly compared using the FPP parameter. This impact on the blood flow may be related to the well-known smooth muscle relaxation induced by dipyrone.

The data presented in this paper show that the analgeic effect of dipyrone can clearly be demonstrated in an experimental psychophysiological study on healthy subjects if the experimental model includes sensitization of peripheral nociceptors and/or secondary neurones.

Acknowledgements

This work was supported by Hoechst AG and by the Deutsche Forschungs-gemeinschaft (grant Ha 831/8).

References

1. H.K. Beecher, Limiting factors in experimental pain. J. chron. Dis. *4*, 11–26 (1953).
2. H.K. Beecher, The measurement of pain. Pharmacol. Rev. *9*, 59–209 (1957).
3. R. Melzack, K.L. Casey, Sensory, motivational, and central control determinants of pain. In «The Skin Senses», (Ed. D. Kenshalo) pp. 423–443, Thomas, Springfield, 1968.
4. H.O. Handwerker, What peripheral mechanims contribute to nociceptive transmission and hyperalgesia? In «Towards a New Pharmacology of Pain – Beyond Morphine», Proceedings of a Dahlem conference. J. Wiley, Chichester, 1990 (in press).
5. F. Anton, H.O. Handwerker, A. Kreh, P. W. Reeh, E. Walter, E. Weber, Influence of acetylsalicylic and salicylic plasma levels on psychophysical measures of long standing natural pain stimuli. In «Advances in Pain Research and Therapy», (Ed. H.L. Fields et al.) pp. 781–789, Raven Press, New York 1985.
6. C. Forster, F. Anton, P.W. Reeh, E. Weber, H.O. Handwerker, Measurement of the analgesic effects of aspirin with a new experimental algesimetric procedure. Pain *32*, 215–222 (1988).
7. H.O. Handwerker, G. Geldner, W. Magerl, Assessment of local skin reactions and of sympathetic vasoconstrictor reflexes with infra-red thermography. Eur. J. Neurosci., Suppl. 2, 168 (1989).

8. I. Martin, P.H. Venables, Techniques in psychophysiology, J. Wiley & Sons, Chichester, 1980.

9. H. Adriaensen, J. Gybels, H.O. Handwerker, J. Van Hees, Nociceptor discharges and sensations during prolonged noxious mechanical stimulation – a paradox. Human Neurobiol. *3*, 53–58 (1984).

Testing the analgesic activity of dipyrone in human subjects using an experimental pain model with tonic and phasic pain stimuli

G. Kobal, H. Huber, E. Pauli and Th. Hummel
Institut für Pharmakologie und Toxikologie
der Universität Erlangen
Universitätsstraße 22
D–8520 Erlangen, F.R.G.

Introduction

The pain-alleviating property of dipyrone has been demonstrated in numerous studies [1]. However, only a small number of approaches try to establish the analgesic action of dipyrone quantitatively by means of experimental pain models [2][3][4]. Even the technique of pain-related evoked potentials, when employed in this field, yielded only unsatisfactory results (reviewed by [5]). It is quite conceivable that this is due to the fact that in most cases phasic painful stimuli were used without an actual inflammatory process being present. Under such conditions the non-steroidal anti-inflammatory drugs (NSAIDs), in particular, are able to develop only a small part of their analgesic efficacy.

In contrast with animal experiments, in human experimentation ethical considerations prohibit the induction of severe inflammatory processes. The aim of the present study was to find out, whether by presenting tolerably painful tonic stimuli – in connection with phasic stimuli this problem could be solved and whether it would consequently be possible to obtain quantitative and objective data on the analgesic action of dipyrone. At the moment we are able to report several successfully performed studies, in which such a combined pain model has been employed in order to investigate the peripherally acting analgesics keto-profen and ibuprofen (Hummel et al. unpublished).

Materials and Methods

Study Design

Five healthy, informed volunteers (4 male, 1 female, between 26 and 36 years of age; mean age 30.2 years) participated in the experiments. A controlled, ran-domized, single blind, two-fold crossover study design was chosen with a washout phase of at least one week in between the drug administrations. The minutes of the experiments were examined and approved by the Ethics Committee of the University of Erlangen-Nürnberg. Each subject participated in two experimental sessions, in which either placebo (0.9% NaCl) or 1 g of dipyrone (Novalgin®) was intravenously administered by infusion using an indwelling catheter (30 min., 250 ml 0.9% NaCl solution). Each experimental session consisted of three 30-min. measuring sequences. The first sequence commenced before and the others 35 and 120 min. after administration of the trial medication. On the day preceding the actual experiment, subjects were requested to attend an adaptation session, in which they became aquainted with all the details appertaining to the study and the experimental procedure.

The Pain Model

In order to present *phasic* painful stimuli a stimulator was used which allowed the application of carbon-dioxide stimuli (CO_2) to the nasal mucosa without simultaneously altering the mechanical or thermal conditions at this site [6]. This monomodal chemical stimulation was achieved in such a way that non-odorous CO_2 was admixed to a carrier gas (air), while the flow rate (145 ml/sec) and temperature (22° C) remained constant. The maximum concentration of a stimulus at the stimulator's outlet was reached within 20 msec. Stimulus duration was 200 msec. Three different stimulus intensities were chosen (45, 52 and 58% v/v CO_2).

In order to attain a *tonic* painful stimulation, a stream of dry air was conducted into the nostril throughout the entire measuring sequence, starting five minutes before the beginning of the experiment. Subjects reported a dull or a burning pain. As a rule, the slight swelling induced by this procedure as a result of a mild, controlled inflammation, as well as the pain at the nasal mucosa decreased and eased off immediately after termination of the experiment, and both disappeared completely whithin one hour. The phasic CO_2 stimuli applied during the measuring sequences were clearly distinguishable from the continuous, tonic pain.

In order to rule out any circulation of air inside the nasal cavity due to breathing, which might have altered the applied stimuli in an uncontrollable manner, the subjects practised a specific kind of respiration acquired during the adaptational session: breathing through the mouth, they placed the soft palate against the posterior pharyngeal wall and thus completely closed the nasal cavity at the back (velopharyngeal closure, [6]).

The experimental parameters were: estimates of painful intensities (intensity estimates of the phasic CO_2 stimuli and of the tonic pain), the mastering of a task for checking vigilance (tracking performance), chemical somatosensory evoked potentials (CSSEP), frequency spectra of the spontaneous EEG, acoustic evoked potentials (AEP), and side effects.

I. Estimates of painful intensities

a)   Estimates of the tonic CO_2 stimuli: 3–4 seconds after presentation of a stimulus, the subjects estimated the intensity of the tonic painful stimulus, i.e. they compared the actually perceived stimulus intensity with the intensity of a standard stimulus, which had been presented at the beginning of the experiment. Subjects estimated the painful intensity of the stimuli by employing a visual analogue scale displayed on a computer screen. This assessment of intensity estimates followed the technique of cross modality matching with prescribed modulus.

b)   Intensity estimates of the tonic painful stimulation: using a similar procedure as described in (a), the subjects reported the intensity of the actual, perceived tonic painful stimuli 12 times during one measuring sequence. On the same computer screen, the extremes of the visual analogue scale were now differently defined, with the left and right extremes corresponding to the verbal expressions of «no painful sensation» and «intolerably strong pain», respectively.

II. Tracking performance

In order to observe changes in the subjects' state of vigilance (and/or motorial co-ordination) they were requested to perform a simple task on a video screen; they had to keep a smaller square, which could be controlled by a joy-stick, inside a larger square which was moving around unpredictably. This «tracking perform-ance» was checked by counting how often, and by measuring for how long, they lost track of the independently moving square.

III. EEG parameters

Pain-related changes in the electroencephalogram (EEG) were recorded as chemosomatosensory evoked potentials (CSSEP). The EEG was recorded from 7 positions of the 10/20 system referenced to linked earlobes (A1+A2). From an additional site (Fp2/A1+A2) possible blink artifacts were registered. For recording, silver-silverchlorided electrodes (2.5 mm^2) were used. The band pass of the system was between 0.2 and 70 Hz and the sampling frequency of the stimulus-linked EEG segments (2048 msec.) was 250 Hz. Recording started 540 msec. before stimulus onset. The mean value of the pre-stimulus period served as baseline for amplitude measurements. The EEG segments were digitized and stored on magnetic media in a computer (PDP11/23, DEC). Data were evaluated off-line using the OFFLAB [6] and POLLUX programs (Schneider and Kobal, unpublished). All single responses contaminated by eye blinks or eye movements were discarded from the average, and averaged responses with a blink artifact greater than 40 µV in the Fp2 lead (Fp2/A1+A2) were excluded from further analysis [7]. Using the same techniques, late near-field acoustic evoked potentials (AEP) were recorded in order to detect unspecific cortical effects of the medication (20 stimuli 5 kHz bursts of 300 msec., 105 dB HL, randomly applied during the intervals between phasic painful stimuli). With a sampling frequency of 125 Hz, the pre-stimulus segments (4096 msec.) were recorded by an IBM/AT-compatible computer. After examining them for blink or motor artifacts, they were submitted to frequency analysis (Fast Fourier Transformation, FFT). The power spectra were averaged in the same way as the post-stimulus records. Subsequently, they were divided into 7 frequency bands (delta 1–3.5 Hz, theta 3.5–7 Hz, alpha1 7–10 Hz, alpha2 10–13 Hz, beta1 13–18 Hz, beta2 18–21 Hz, beta3 21–30 Hz). The integrated power of the bands was used for further statistical evaluation [8].

IV. Side effects

All reports given by the subjects during the experiments were noted down. Additionally, visual analogue scales were given to the subjects after termination of each measuring sequence, in which they were requested to indicate the intensity of the following symptoms: drowsiness («Müdigkeit»), dizziness («Benommen-heit»), discharge of nasal mucuous secretion, vertigo («Schwindel»), sensation of cold and headache.

V. Vital parameters

Prior to and during the measurements, the heart rate, as well as the systolic and diastolic blood pressure were checked in each subject.

Statistical Evaluation

Data were submitted to analysis of variances (MANOVA) using SPSS PC+ programs with medication and measuring sequences as within-subject factors. If MANOVA results were significant, t-tests were employed.

Results

The results obtained from the after investigation of the evoked potentials (pain-related potentials CSSEP, acoustic evoked potentials AEP) will be reported elsewhere.

    The question as to whether this newly developed pain model is suited for establishing the analgesic action of dipyrone must be answered in the affirmative.

I.   Estimates of painful intensity: Table I gives a survey of most mean values and standard deviations of measured parameters. Fig. 1 clearly shows that after administration of dipyrone, estimates of painful intensity were lower compared to placebo. The differences were statistically significant ($p < 0.07$). It is quite likely that, had more subjects participated, the differences between placebo and dipyrone would have been even more conspicuous. The decrease by approximately 11 EU 30 min. after placebo might have been due to either a placebo effect or momentary habituation. Even at this early stage, an analgesic action of dipyrone could be discerned; 120 min. after administration of the trial medication, when estimates of the tonic painful stimulus were back to their initial level under placebo, the efficacy of dipyrone became evident; estimates of the tonic pain were approximately 20 EU lower under dipyrone (0 EU = no pain, 100 EU = intolerably strong pain).

No placebo effect was found with phasic pain stimuli (Fig. 2). In the course of the investigation, intensity estimates after administration of placebo increased to the same extent as did the intensity estimates of the tonic painful stimuli. After administration of dipyrone, a decrease in estimates could be observed for all three stimulus strengths, which was particularly pronounced in the very strong stimuli (58% v/v CO_2).

II.   There were no statistically significant differences in the tracking performances after administration of either placebo or dipyrone (Fig. 3).

III.   The results of the frequency analysis of the spontaneous EEG revealed a marked decrease in the low frequency bands (delta and theta) as early as 30 min. after administration of dipyrone, as compared with placebo (Fig. 4). All other frequency bands were virtually unaltered. This kind of decrease clearly indicated an increase in arousal.

IV.   Consistent with the results of the frequency analyses, the subjects reported feeling less drowsy after administration of dipyrone than after placebo (Fig. 3).

V.   A vasodilative action of dipyrone, frequently claimed in the literature [9], was only observed in the form of a momentary drop in blood pressure which was evidently already compensated by an increase in heart rate (Fig. 5). These findings were also statistically significant when compared to placebo.

Discussion

The present study was able to prove the suitability of an experimental pain model – which provides tonic, as well as phasic painful stimuli – for establishing the analgesic action of dipyrone, even if only a small number of subjects is investigated. The combination of the experimental parameters revealed that besides its analgesic properties, dipyrone most probably also has an effect on the central nervous system. It is interesting to note that the analgesia which dipyrone produces

[min. after administration]		Placebo				Dipyrone			
		-30	30	120	150	-30	30	120	150
Nasal Secretion	M:	20.0	18.6	20.0		22.3	11.1	11.8	
	SD:	16.7	18.4	16.9		29.8	3.9	11.0	
Drowsiness	M:	7.5	23.2	16.2		23.9	10.1	1.9	
	SD:	11.8	22.2	26.1		30.3	18.7	2.9	
Tracking Performance	M:	73.5	75.9	77.9		74.5	77.0	78.6	
	SD:	6.0	5.1	3.8		4.3	5.6	5.4	
Estimates: Phasic Pain 45% v/v CO_2	M:	30.6	31.2	43.1		38.9	45.1	43.0	
	SD:	18.2	18.9	24.4		16.2	12.6	19.8	
52% v/v CO_2	M:	48.6	50.8	58.9		63.0	75.4	63.8	
	SD:	10.7	30.7	21.4		16.2	7.4	21.4	
58% v/v CO_2	M:	67.8	68.2	69.4		90.3	97.0	80.7	
	SD:	31.8	38.9	18.4		6.8	15.5	24.3	
Estimates: Tonic Pain	M:	38.7	27.8	39.2		51.4	32.3	35.1	
	SD:	24.4	21.9	24.6		19.8	24.8	16.8	
Frequency Analysis Pos. Fz: delta Band	M:	323	338	338		351	328	342	
	SD:	40	31	23		35	28	20	
Pos. Fz: theta Band	M:	333	374	374		346	360	342	
	SD:	61	67	43		63	52	36	
Pos. Pz: delta Band	M:	310	321	320		339	326	319	
	SD:	55	51	43		40	39	33	
Pos. Pz: theta Band	M:	289	308	307		308	310	306	
	SD:	54	56	44		45	38	37	
Heart Rate	M:	79.4	67.6	77.6	68.6	69.2	69.2	72.6	67.2
	SD:	19.0	15.6	11.5	13.5	19.8	13.2	9.7	8.2
Arterial Blood Pressure	M:	117.2	119.6	127.2	120.0	120.0	116.8	120.4	118.8
	SD:	20.1	20.9	18.2	17.8	18.0	14.4	7.4	11.1
Diastolic Blood Pressure	M:	68.4	70.6	74.8	69.4	74.2	72.8	74.8	74.6
	SD:	15.6	15.9	7.3	9.5	15.0	9.6	2.6	8.1

Tab. 1.
Means (M) and standard deviations (SD) of experimental parameters.
[Heart rate in beats per minute, blood pressure in mm Hg; ratings in estimation units; tracking performance in U; results of frequency analyses in arbitrary units]

is not linked with the sedative effect usually observed with analgesics that act on the central nervous system (such as opioids), but rather with central stimulation. This was deduced from the fact that the power of the low-frequency parts of the spontaneous EEG decreased, which coincided with a subjectively less intensely experienced drowsiness as compared with placebo. With respect to phasic painful stimuli it may be assumed that, in combination with tonic painful stimuli, the intensity estimates were far more sensitive in indicating the action of peripherally acting analgesics than when used on their own. The reason for this might be the mild inflammation momentarily induced by the tonic painful stimuli, which led to a more pronounced sensitization when the analgesic was not administered.

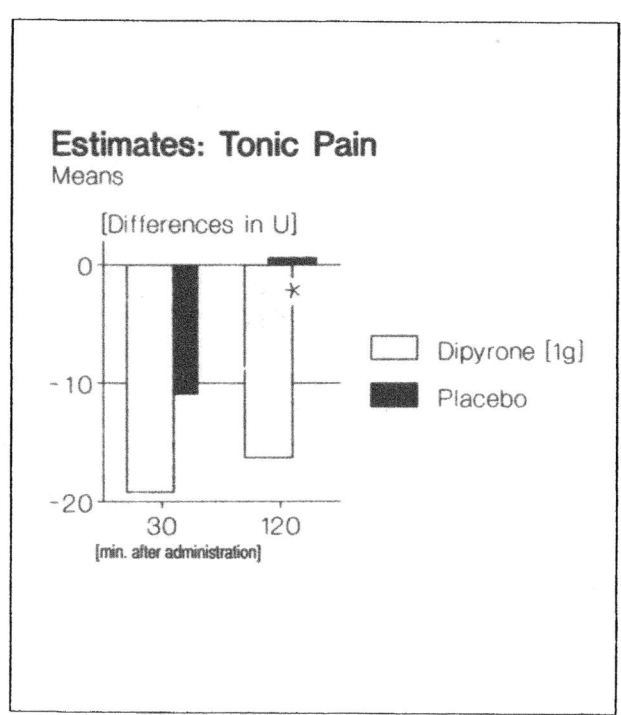

Fig. 1.
Mean differences between pre- and postmedication values of intensity estimates of the tonic pain stimulation. 0 U = no pain, 100 U = intolerably strong pain. 120 min. after administration of dipyrone, estimates are considerably lower than after administration of placebo (* = p<0.07).

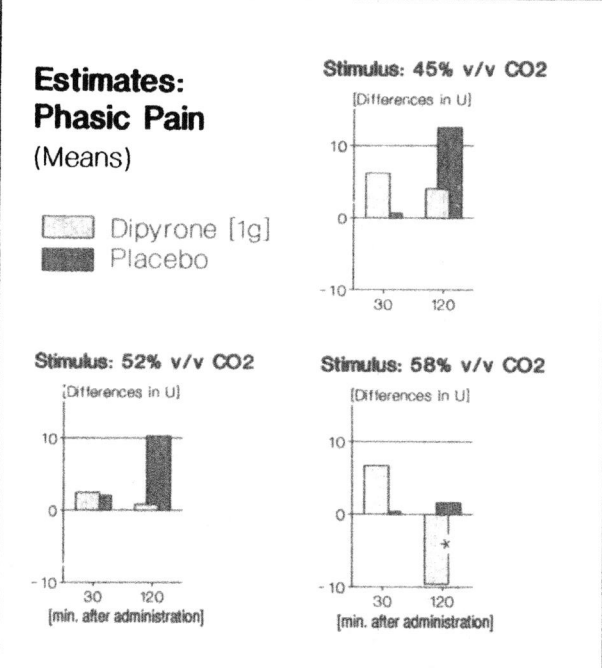

Fig. 2.
Mean differences between pre- and postmedication values of intensity estimates of the phasic pain stimuli. 0 U = no pain, 100 U = intensity of the standard pain stimulus, which was applied as the first stimulus in the experiment before drug administration (52% v/v CO_2). 120 min. after administration of dipyrone, estimates are considerably lower than after administration of placebo.

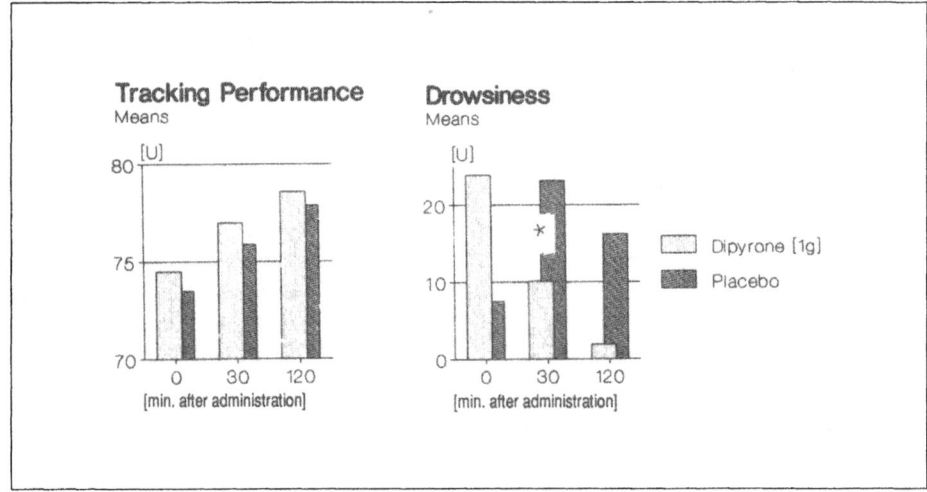

Fig. 3.
Mean values of tracking performance and estimates of drowsiness. Tracking Perfomance: 0
U = no succesful tracking at all, 100 U = best tracking performance. Drowsiness: 0 U = very
alert, 100 U = very tired. General improvement in the tracking performance is due to learning
effects. Subjects feel less tired after administration of dipyrone (* = p<0.08).

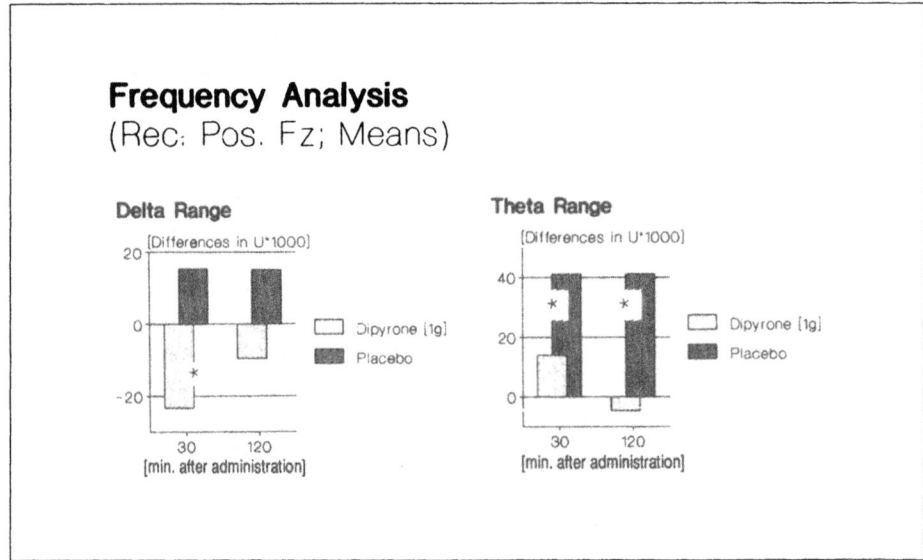

Fig. 4.
Mean differences between pre- and postmedication values of the power densities in the delta
and theta ranges. Recording position Fz. Administration of dipyrone reduces power densities
in the delta frequency band indicating arousal of the subject (* = p<0.05).

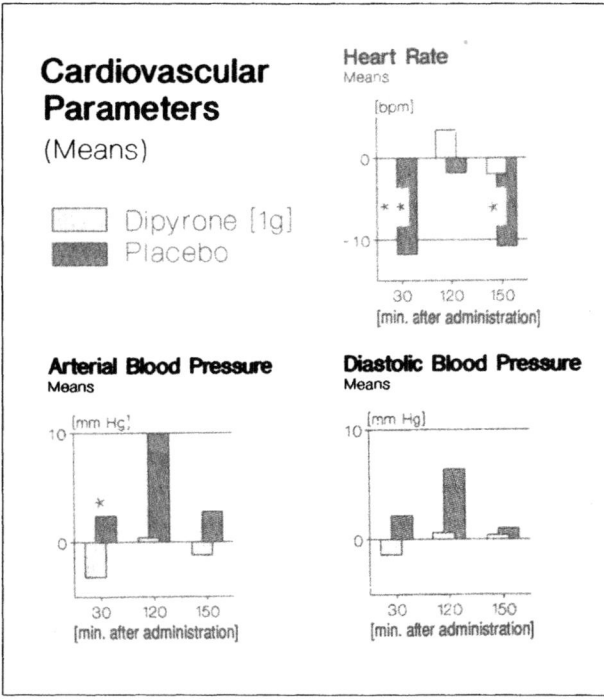

Fig. 5.
Mean differences between pre- and postmedication values of systolic and diastolic blood pressure, and heart rate (* = p<0.1; ** = p<0.05).

References

1. Brune K (ed.): 100 years of pyrazolone drugs. Agents and Actions Suppl. *19* (1986).
2. Kobal G, Raab E: The effect of analgesics on pain-related somatosensory evoked potentials, Agents and Actions Suppl. *19* (1986) 75–88.
3. Rohdewald P, Drehsen G, Milsmann E, Derendorf H: Relationship between saliva levels of metamizol metabolites, bioavailability and analgesic efficacy. Arzneim. Forsch. Drug Res. *33*(II)7 (1983) 985–988.
4. Handwerker HO, Beck A, Forster C, Gall Th, Magerl W, this volume.
5. Kobal G, Hummel C, Nuernberg B, Brune K: Effects of Pentazocine and Acetylsalicylic Acid on Pain-rating and Vigilance in Relationship to Pharmacokinetic Parameters. Agents and Actions *29* (1990) 342–359.
6. Kobal G: Elektrophysiologische Untersuchungen des menschlichen Geruchssinnes. Thieme, Stuttgart (1981).
7. Kobal G, Hummel C: Cerebral chemosensory evoked potentials elicited by chemical stimulation of the human olfactory and respiratory nasal mucosa. Electroenceph. clin. Neurophysiol. *71* (1988) 241–250.
8. Kobal G, Hummel Th: Effects of flupirtine on the pain-related evoked potential and the spontaneous EEG. Agents and Actions *23* 1/2 (1988) 117–119.
9. Zoppi M, Hoigne R, Keller MF, Streit F, Hess T: Blutdruckabfall unter Dipyron (Novaminsulfon-Natrium). Schweiz. med. Wschr. *113* (1983) 1768–1770.

Unwanted drug effects of antipyretic analgesics: epidemiological data

M. Levy
Department of Medicine A, Hadassah University Hospital
Jerusalem, 91120, Israel

During the eighties, the antipyretic analgesic drugs continued to fulfil the human need for pain and fever relief, remaining the most commonly used drugs. In the United States, 1.2 billion dollars were spent in 1980 on analgesic drugs [1]. Three pharmacological drug groups have prevailed throughout the century: the salicylates, para-aminophenols and the pyrazolone derivatives.

Still, several important changes have occurred on the analgesic antipyretics utilization and regulation scene of the past decade. Paracetamol (acetaminophen), the major metabolite of phenacetin, has replaced aspirin as the most commonly used drug, available almost everywhere as an over-the-counter drug, while phenacetin – a prime culprit for analgesic nephropathy – practically disappeared, however without the expected answer to the disease. Aspirin has changed feathers; it has become a leading cardiovascular drug due to its effect on platelet aggregation. Its use as an analgesic antipyretic in children and adolescents became illadvised because of the risk of Reye's syndrome. Amidopyrine, the veteran pyrazolone derivative, is no longer in use because of its potential carcinogenicity. In animals it leads to the formation of nitrosamines. Dipyrone continued, in some countries, to be the number one analgesic antipyretic available over the counter whilst in others it was banned. Its use remained the centre of pharmacopolitical debates, often divorced from pharmacoepidemiology.

The most important discovery of the decade regarding the adversities of the analgesic antipyretic drugs has no doubt been aspirin's role in Reye's syndrome. This discovery indeed resulted in a marked decrease in the incidence of the disease due to the decreased use of aspirin by the population at risk.

Ten years ago, I summarized an epidemiological evaluation of rare side effects of mild analgesics, concluding that major adverse reactions to these drugs – unless they were abused or taken in high doses – were rare (i.e. the risk to the individual was low). However, because of the massive and universal use of these drugs, quantitative measurement of the risk (i.e. public health hazard) involved is imperative, and it is only by conducting epidemiological studies that data leading to decisions based on scientifically sound judgements may be obtained [2].

In the following, I shall attempt to review some of the relevant studies performed during the decade, so as to give examples from my own experience and to provide, whenever available, the current quantitative estimate of risk of analgesic antipyretic drug-induced hepatotoxicity, nephropathy, haematological reactions, gastrointestinal reactions and allergic and pseudoallergic reactions. Emphasis will be placed on the importance of estimating excess risk (i.e. attributable risk or absolute risk or incidence), namely the number of cases per defined number of persons exposed to a defined dose for a certain length of exposure, and the aetiological fraction (i.e., the proportion of the disease attributable to the use of a specific drug).

Hepatotoxicity

In line with being a most common household remedy, the incidence of paracetamol poisoning is on the increase. In Jerusalem, the incidence of hospital referrals for paracetamol overdosage went up from 0.5 per 100,000 inhabitants in 1978 to 4.5 per 100,000 in 1983 [3] and to about 10 per 100,000 in 1988. In the U.S. and the U.K. paracetamol poisoning was estimated to account for 50% of the total number of drug poisonings [4]. In the U.K. paracetamol poisoning appears to be the most common cause of acute liver failure [5]. Our experience in Jerusalem in terms of hepatotoxicity from paracetamol overdosage has been that morbidity was low because of the availability of diagnostic and therapeutic measures. During a recent measles epidemic we noted that disturbances in liver function tests were more common in those treated for fever with paracetamol compared to those who were given dipyrone [6].

Aspirin hepatotoxicity is also dose-related. Young females with conditions such as rheumatic fever and juvenile rheumatic arthritis seem to carry a higher risk [7]. The magnitude of the risk of clinically relevant hepatotoxicity in aspirin users is unknown. Transient elevations of liver enzymes were reported in half the patients given full anti-inflammatory doses of aspirin [8]. Dipyrone does not appear to cause hepatotoxicity [9].

Reye's syndrome

The first case-control study showing an association between Reye's syndrome and salicylates in children with antecedent viral illness, mainly influenza and chicken pox, appeared in 1980 [10]. This was followed by three additional case-report studies, published in 1982 [11][12]. In all these studies, a strong association was found and more than 95% of the cases were exposed to salicylates. Still, criticism was raised about the methods used and questions asked concerning selection and misclassification bias. Eventually, a new study was undertaken by the (U.S.)

Public Health Service task force on Reye's syndrome. In the pilot, as well as in the main study published in 1987 [13][14], a clear-cut association was found with exposure of salicylates during the antecedent illness (chicken pox, respiratory or gastrointestinal illness) prior to the onset of Reye's syndrome. The rate ratio was 40 (lower 95% confidence limit: 5.8) for salicylates as a group and 26 (6.4) for aspirin.

In 1985 when aspirin use in children was already on the decline, only 91 of Reye's syndrome cases were reported to the U.S. Centers for Disease Control compared to 1003 cases during the years 1981 through 1985.

It is evident that salicylates play an aetiological role in the majority of cases of Reye's syndrome (aetiological fraction >90%). The intriguing question as to why it occurs particularly with chickenpox and influenza in children and adolescents remains to be answered. In all studies, no association was found between paracetamol use and Reye's syndrome.

Analgesic nephropathy

Analgesic nephropathy is characterized by papillary necrosis and chronic tubular interstitial disease. There appears to be a marked geographical variation in the incidence of the disease. Between 1% and 30% of uremic patients were found to be excessive analgesic consumers [15]. It constitutes the most common drug-related chronic renal disease. Dubach et al. [16] in their 11-year follow-up study found that women using phenacetin-containing analgesics, compared to a control group, had higher serum creatinine levels and both overall and renal and urogenital mortality rates. McCredie et al. [17] in their case-control study reported a rate ratio of 18 for the association between phenacetin comsumption and papillary necrosis. Sandler et al. [18] recently reported that daily users of analgesics had significantly more renal disease than infrequent users. The rate ratio after adjustment for the effects of other analgesics was highest in daily users of phenacetin (5.1, lower 95% confidence limit: 1.7). For daily paracetamol users the rate was 3.2 (1.05). Rate ratios with daily and weekly use of aspirin-phenacetin-caffeine mixtures were also significantly elevated. However, no association was found between daily aspirin use (after adjustment for the effects of other analgesics) and renal disease. The risk associated with phenacetin increased with the cummulative dose. Stratified by the type of renal disease, it was highest for interstitial nephritis. This study, although leaving many questions open, is important because it lends further support to the Australian experience that restriction of phenacetin by itself did not result in the expected reduction in the incidence of analgesic nephropathy [19]. However, restriction of the sales of analgesic mixtures containing combinations of aspirin, phenacetin, paracetamol, salicylamide and caffeine seems to be effective.

Still, today, 37 years after analgesic nephropathy was first described by Spuhler and Zollinger [20], many questions remain open. What is the role in nephropathy of aspirin, a drug convincingly shown in experiments done by Kincaid-Smith and her group to cause papillary necrosis, and what is the excess risk for the various drug combinations?

There have been several case-report studies and one recent cohort study [21] describing an association between analgesic use and cancer of the renal pelvis or renal cell carcinoma. Once again, none of these studies provides estimates of the excess risk. The issue certainly deserves more scrutiny.

Haematological reactions

There have been case-reports of haemolytic anaemia in people with glucose 6-phosphate dehydrogenase deficiency exposed to aspirin and paracetamol. Dipyrone also, without any evidence, appears on textbook lists of drugs causing that condition. At present the causal role of all the analgesic antipyretic drugs in this type of haemolytic anaemia is not substantiated.

It comes as no surprise that all analgesic antipyretic drugs have been reported to cause agranulocytosis. All such drugs would appear in the drug histories of patients with agranulocytosis because fever and pain are the initial symptoms of the disease [22]. The causal relationship between pyrazolone derivatives and agranulocytosis has long been established [23]. Still, in most reports multiple drugs that could potentially cause the disease were given and judgements as to the offending drug tended to be made according to a prior suspicion rather than scientific criteria.

Attempts in the sixties and the seventies to quantify the risk were unsatisfactory and regulatory decisions about the use of pyrazolone derivates were not substantiated by scientific data. This situation led to the first analytical epidemiological study of the drug aetiology of agranulocytosis and aplastic anaemia – the International Agranulocytosis and Aplastic Anaemia Study (IAAAS).

The methods used in this population-based case-control study were published in 1983 [24] and a first report on analgesics followed in 1986 [25]. In that study, analgesic antipyretic drug use in the week before the clinical onset of illness, i.e. the period of aetiological significance, was compared between 221 confirmed cases of agranulocytosis and 1425 hospital controls identified by the study centres in Jerusalem, Berlin, Ulm, Milan, Barcelona, Sofia, Budapest and Stockholm. The study base comprised the total experience in these areas during the 1980–1984 period, which amounted to close on 80 million person-years.

For salicylates the multivariate rate ratio (relative risk) estimate was 1.6, but of borderline statistical significance (lower 95% confidence limit: 1.0). For paracetamol, no association was found (rate ratio: 1.0). There was a significant regional variability in the rate ratio estimate for the use of dipyrone. In Ulm, Berlin and Barcelona (grouped together) it was 23.7 (lower 95% c.l.: 8.7), for Israel (1980–1986) 2.0 (0.9). In Budapest and Sofia the estimates were close to unity, in Milan data were too sparse, while in Stockholm dipyrone was not in use. The aetiological fraction for dipyrone use in Ulm, Berlin and Barcelona amounted to 27%, and the excess risk estimate in those regions connected with hospital admission for agranulocytosis from any dipyrone use in a seven-day period amounted to 1.1 cases per million users.

The reason for the geographical variation in the risk of dipyrone-induced agranulocytosis is highly intriguing [26]. Efforts made by the investigators to detect to what extent the variation is a reflection of methodological problems or hidden bias have not provided an answer. If real, regional differences could provide an important scientific lead in understanding the aetiology of the disease [27].

In the IAAAS, analgesic use 29 to 180 days before admission was also compared between 113 cases of aplastic anaemia and 1724 controls. For the use of salicylates on four or more days in any week, the rate ratio estimate was 2.9; however, this result was not statistically significant. There was no association between paracetamol or dipyrone use and aplastic anaemia.

Case-reports of immune thrombocytopenia in individuals exposed to aspirin and paracetamol have been published [28]. These are rare events and there are no quantitative estimates of risk. Similarly, no quantitative estimates are available as regards the risk of aspirin-related bleeding in patients with conditions such as haemophilia, von Willebrand's disease and hereditary telangiectasia. The issue of gastrointestinal bleeding will be discussed next.

Gastrointestinal complications

The association between aspirin and gastric ulceration and between aspirin and major upper gastrointestinal bleeding became evident from case-control studies done in the sixties and the seventies. None of these studies clearly distinguished whether aspirin use preceded clinical symptoms of the disease. In 1974, we calculated estimates for the association between heavy, regular aspirin use and benign gastric ulcer and major upper gastrointestinal bleeding; we found rate ratios of 2.1 and 3.4 and attributable risks of 10 and 15 cases per 100,000 users per year, respectively [29]. Coggon et al. in 1983 [30] compared aspirin and paracetamol consumption in matched pairs of patients with major upper gastrointestinal bleeding and community controls. Higher rates for both drugs were found in the cases. However, for aspirin the association was found with both recent and habitual use, whereas for paracetamol it was only evident for recent use which could have related to symptoms of the disease. It was indirectly estimated (based on hospital admission rates for major upper gastrointestinal bleeding of 1 in 2000–2500 per year for the general population) that the excess risk for regular aspirin users would amount to 40 per 100,000 per year. It was further estimated that the risk of being admitted for major upper gastrointestinal bleeding was one for every 250,000 aspirin doses.

In both studies drug histories anteceded the day of admission, not the day on which symptoms commenced. It now appears that in our 1974 study we under-estimated both the rate ratio and the overall incidence of bleeding.

More recently, we have used some of the experience gained in the IAAAS for the methods employed in a new case-control study [31]. The risk of a first episode of major upper gastrointestinal bleeding in subjects not known to be predisposed was assessed in relation to the use of analgesics.

For aspirin use during at least four days within the week before the onset of symptoms, the rate ratio estimate was 15 (lower 95% c.l.: 6.4) and for occasional use, 5.6 (2.7). There was no evidence that paracetamol use increased the risk. Although the methods used in this study do not allow estimation of excess risk, our results suggest that the risk for aspirin users is substantially higher than previously thought. From epidemilogical studies on recipients of non-aspirin non-steroidal anti-inflammatory drugs (NSAIDs), a doubling to quadrupling of the risk of ulcer complications is suggested. The risk appears to be increasing with age [32].

As some of these drugs are now available over the counter (OTC) and used as analgesics-antipyretics, the risks of OTC non-aspirin NSAID-related and aspirin-related gastrointestinal bleeding (as well as agranulocytosis, aplastic anaemia, etc.) are of concern and should be further evaluated, particularly in the elderly. The clinical impression is that dipyrone use is not associated with gastrointestinal bleeding. This should be corroborated by epidemilogical data.

Allergic and pseudo-allergic reactions

Epidemilogical evaluation is still almost entirely lacking for these potentially life-threatening conditions. Anaphylactic and anaphylactoid reactions, including laryngeal and angioneurotic oedema, generalized urticaria, bronchospasm, vaso-motor collapse and death, have been described, in particular after parenteral injection of pyrazolone derivatives and NSAIDs. Kewitz et al. [33] reported that the risk associated with pyrazolone derivatives is not higher than that with opioids. Aspirin hypersensitivity is more common in people with asthma, nasal polyps, rhinitis and chronic urticaria. It may cross-react with pyrazolone derivatives and

NSAIDs [34]. Dipyrone-induced skin rashes are relatively frequent and the specific drug aetiology is often missed [35].

In summary, some progress was made during the decade in the pharmacoepidemiological research on the adverse effects to analgesic antipyretic drugs. For some of the important events such as gastrointestinal bleeding and agranulocytosis, quantitative estimates became available. Unfortunately, pharmacopolitical considerations have not always guaranteed scientifically-based regulatory actions. Unnecessary delays occurred while unveiling the drug aetiology of Reye's syndrome. Nevertheless, the story of Reye's syndrome exemplified the importance and potential of epidemiological research.

Major adverse reactions to analgesics-antipyretics are still to be considered rare, but aspirin-induced gastrointestinal bleeding appears to be more common than previously thought and may also occur after occasional use.

There are still fascinating questions to be answered concerning the aetiology and pathogenesis of these adverse events. For a reaction occurring once in a million exposures (sometimes in individuals with a history of frequent use in the past without adversity) a multifactorial aetiology has to be considered.

In Reye's syndrome, combined effects of drug use and viral infection seem to operate, and we have some hints that this might also be true for dipyrone-induced agranulocytosis [36]. Other factors such as genetic or environment-related predisposition are suggested by the geographical variation in the incidence of some of the reactions.

Answers to these questions, the identification of subpopulations carrying higher risks and the availability of comparable quantitative data for all major adverse events to analgesic antipyretic drugs should be goals for the end of the century.

References

1. Consumer expenditure study: internal analgesics. Product Marketing and Cosmetical Fragrance Retailing. *10*:38, 1981.
2. Levy, M., Epidemiological evaluation of rare side-effects of mild analgesics. Br. J. Clin. Pharmacol. *10*:395S–399S, 1980.
3. Levy, M., Oren, R., Paracetamol overdosage in Jerusalem. 1978–1983. Isr. J. Med. Sci. *21*:36–39, 1985.
4. Paulozzi, L.J., Seasonality of reported poison exposures. Pediatrics. *71*:891–893, 1983.
5. Meredith, T. J., and Vale, J.A., Non-narcotic analgesics: Problems of overdosage. Drugs *32* (suppl. 4), 177–205, 1986.
6. Ackerman, Z., Flugelman, M., Wax, J., et al., Hepatitis during measles in young adults: Possible role of antipyretic drugs. Hepatology, 1990 (in press).
7. Zimmerman, H.J., Effects of aspirin and paracetamol on the liver. Arch. Intern. Med. *141*:333–342, 1981.

8. Prescott, L.F., Effects of non-narcotic analgesics on the liver. Drugs *32* (suppl. 4), 129–147, 1986.
9. Vanacek, J., Antipyretic analgesics. In: Dukes M.N.G. (Ed.). Side effects of drugs. Elsevier. Amsterdam 1985, pp. 75–82.
10. Starko, K.M., Ray, C.G., Dominguez, L.B., et al., Reye's syndrome and salicylate use. Pediatrics *66*:859–864, 1980.
11. Waldman, P.J., Hall, W.N., McGee, H., et al., Aspirin as a risk factor in Reye's syndrome. JAMA *247*:3089–3094, 1982.
12. Halpin, T.J., Holtzhauer, F.J., Campbell, R.J., et al., Reye's syndrome and medication use. JAMA *248*:687–691, 1982.
13. Hurwitz, E.S., Barret, M.J., Bergman, D., et al., Public Health Service study on Reye's syndrome and medications. Report of the pilot phase. N. Engl. J. Med. *313*:847–857, 1985.
14. Hurwitz, E.S., Barret, M.J., Bregman, D., et al., Public Health Service. Study of Reye's syndrome and medications: The main study. JAMA *257*:1905–1911, 1987.
15. Schreiner, G.E., Chronic drug nephrotoxicity. In: Haddad and Winchester (Eds.). Clinical management of poisoning and drug overdosage. W.B. Saunders, Philadelphia, 1983, pp. 185–197.
16. Dubach, U.C., Rosner, B., Pfister, E., Epidemiologic study of abuse of analgesics containing phenacetin. Renal morbidity and mortality (1968–1979). N. Engl. J. Med. *308*:357–362, 1983.
17. McCredie, M., Steward, J.H., Mahony, J.F., Is phenacetin responsible for analgesic nephropathy in New South Wales? Clin. Nephrol. *17*:134–140, 1982.
18. Sandler, D.P., Smith, J.C., Weinberg, C.R., et al., Analgesic use and chronic renal disease. N. Engl. J. Med. *320*:1238–1243, 1989.
19. Kincaid-Smith, P., Renal toxicity of non-narcotic analgesics. Medical Toxicology *1*: (Suppl. 1) 14–22, 1986.
20. Spuhler, O., Zollinger, H.U., Die chronisch interstitielle Nephritis. Zeitschrift Klinischer Medizin *151*:1–50, 1953.
21. Paganini-Hill, A., Chao, A., Ross, R.K., et al., Aspirin use and chronic diseases: a cohort study of the elderly. Brit. Med. J. *299*:1247–1250, 1989.
22. Levy, M., Causes of agranulocytosis in a hospital population. Identification of dipyrone as an important causative agent? Isr. J. Med. Sci. *19*:110, 1983.
23. Moeschlin, S., and Wagner, K., Agranulocytosis due to the occurrence of leukocyte agglutinins. Acta Haematol. *8*:29, 1952.
24. International Agranulocytosis and Aplastic Anemia Study. Risks of Agranulocytosis and Aplastic Anemia. A first report of their relation to drug use with special reference to analgesics. JAMA *256*:1749–1757, 1986.
25. International Agranulocytosis and Aplastic Anemia Study: The design of a study of the drug etiology of agranulocytosis and aplastic anemia. Europ. J. Clin. Pharmacol. *24*:833–836, 1983.
26. Faich, G.A., Analgesic risk and pharmacoepidemiology. JAMA *256*:1788. 1986.
27. Doll, R., Lunde, P.K.M., and Moeschlin, S., Analgesics, agranulocytosis and aplastic anemia. Lancet *1*, 101, 1987.
28. Scheinberg, I.H., Thrombocytopenic reaction to aspirin and acetaminophen. N. Engl. J. Med. *300*:678, 1979.
29. Levy, M., Aspirin use in patients with major upper gastrointestinal bleeding and peptic ulcer disease. N. Engl. J. Med. *290*:1158–1162, 1974.

30. Coggon, D., Langman, M.J.S., and Spiegalhalter, D., Aspirin, paracetamol and haematemesis and melena. Gut 23:340–344, 1982.
31. Levy, M., Miller, D.R., Kaufman, D.W., et al., Major upper gastrointestinal bleeding. Relation to the use of aspirin and other non-narcotic analgesics. Arch. Intern. Med. 148:281–285, 1988.
32. Langman, M.J.S., Epidemiologic evidence on the association between peptic ulceration and antiinflammatory drug use. Gastroenterology 96:640–646, 1989.
33. Kewitz, H., Harter, G., Feldmann, U., et al., Observational cohort study in general practice: Differences and equivalence among analgesics for treatment of colic pain. In: Kewitz, H., Roots, I., Voight, K. (Eds.) Epidemiologic concepts in clinical pharmacology. Springer Verlag, Berlin 1987, pp. 73–86.
34. Szczeklik, A., Analgesics, allergy and asthma. Drugs 32 (Suppl. 4):1480163, 1986.
35. Boston Colloborative Drug Surveillance Program. (Levy, M.). Dipyrone as a cause of drug rashes. Int. J. Epidemiol. 2:167–170, 1973.
36. Levy, M., The combined effect of viruses and drugs in drug induced diseases. Medical Hypothesis 14:293–294, 1984.